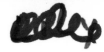

NATURAL WORLD

WOLF

HABITATS • LIFE CYCLES • FOOD CHAINS • THREATS

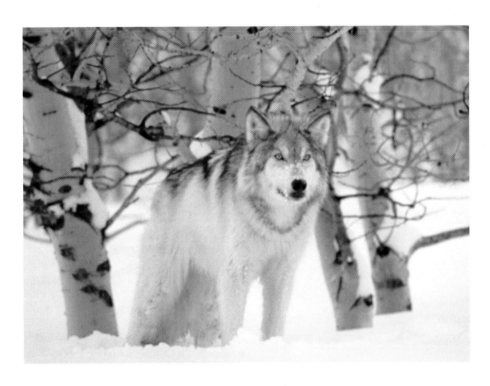

Michael Leach

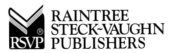
RAINTREE
STECK-VAUGHN
PUBLISHERS

A Harcourt Company

Austin   New York
www.raintreesteckvaughn.com

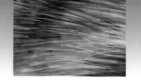

NATURAL WORLD

Black Rhino • Chimpanzee • Crocodile • Dolphin • Elephant • Giant Panda
Giraffe • Golden Eagle • Gorilla • Great White Shark • Grizzly Bear
Hippopotamus • Killer Whale • Koala • Leopard • Lion • Orangutan
Penguin • Polar Bear • Tiger • Wolf • Zebra

Cover: A gray wolf, up close.
Title page: Wolves living in the far north have extra-thick fur to keep out the cold.
Contents page: The wolf is one of the world's shyest and most elusive creatures.
Index page: Wolves can howl at any time of the day, but they are at their noisiest at sunset.

Published by Raintree Steck-Vaughn Publishers,
an imprint of Steck-Vaughn Company

Library of Congress Cataloging-in-Publication data

Leach, Michael.
  Wolf / Michael Leach.
    p. cm. — (Natural world)
  Includes bibliographical references (p.).
  Summary: Describes the physical characteristics, behavior, habitat, and life cycle of wolves, as well as the threats they face and efforts to protect them.
  ISBN 0-7398-5231-0
  1. Wolves—Juvenile literature. [1. Wolves.] I. Title. II. Natural world (Austin, Tex.)

QL737.C22 L43 2002
599.773—dc21   2001048371

Printed in Italy. Bound in the United States.
1 2 3 4 5 6 7 8 9 0 LB 06 05 04 03 02

Picture acknowledgments
Ardea 6 Ferrero/Labat, 10 M Watson, 12 Jean-Paul Ferrero, 13 M Watson, 15 M Watson, 17 M Watson, 22 S Meyers, 25 S Meyers, 39 Eric Dragesco, 44 top M Watson; *Bruce Coleman Collection* front cover, 24 Erwin & Peggy Bauer, 27 Stephen J Krasemann, 48 Erwin & Peggy Bauer; *Corbis* 23 Tom Brakefield, 37 Darrell Gulin, 40 Layne Kennedy, 43 Layne Kennedy, 45 bottom Layne Kennedy; *FLPA* 7 Mark Newman, 9 Yossi Eshbol, 11 Michael Callan, 19 Minden Pictures, 20 Gerard Lacz, 21 Minden Pictures, 26 Mark Newman, 28 W Wisniewski, 29 Minden Pictures, 30 T Whittaker, 31 Minden Pictures, 32 Minden Pictures, 32-3 Minden Pictures, 36 Minden Pictures, 41 Panda/ A Bardi, 44 bottom Gerard Lacz, 45 top Minden Pictures, 45 middle T Whittaker; *Fortean Picture Library* 38; *Michael Leach* 3; *NHPA* 1 John Shaw, 8 John Shaw, 14 Andy Rouse, 16 David Middleton, 18 Andy Rouse, 35 John Shaw, 42 Stephen J Krasemann, 44 middle Andy Rouse. Artwork by Michael Posen.

Contents

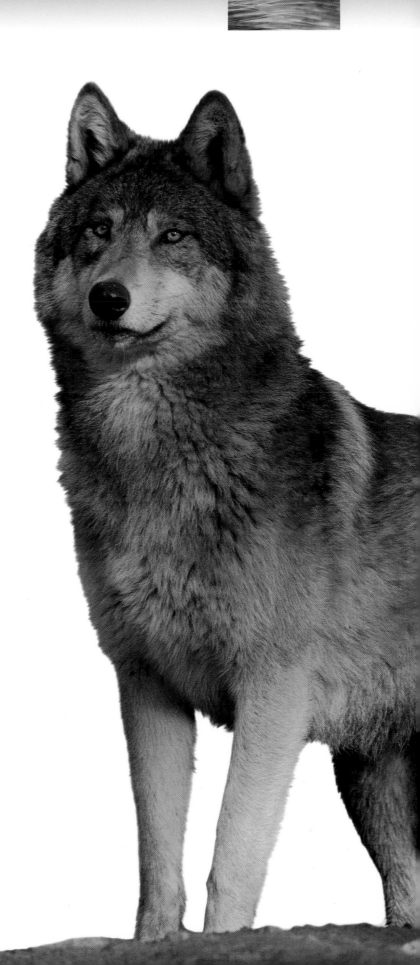

Meet the Wolf

Gray wolves are long-legged members of the dog family that live together in packs. They are mainly meat-eaters, and they are quite intelligent. Gray wolves once lived in many northern parts of the world, but terrible over-hunting by people has greatly reduced their numbers.

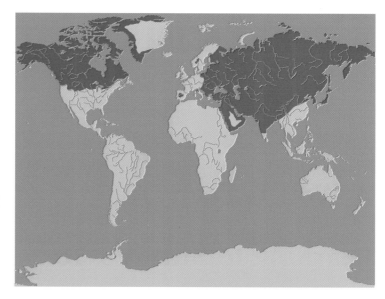

▲ The red shading on this map shows where gray wolves live.

WOLF FACTS

A full-grown adult gray wolf measures up to 34 inches (86 cm) tall at the shoulder, and 6.5 feet (2 meters) in length from nose to tail. It weighs up to 145 pounds (65 kg). Male wolves are larger than females.

●

The scientific name for the gray wolf is *Canis lupus*.

●

Gray wolves are the largest members of the dog family, *Canidae*. There are 35 species in the family, including wild dogs such as coyotes, dingoes, and African hunting dogs, as well as many types of foxes and several kinds of jackals.

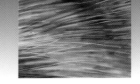

Ears
Large ears pick up the slightest sounds, and are especially useful at night. The ears can turn and swivel to detect sounds from different directions.

Nose
The wolf's long, sensitive nose provides an incredibly keen sense of smell. Wolves can follow the scent of prey more than half a mile (one kilometer) away.

Fur coat
The coat is long and furry. In winter it becomes even thicker, to keep out the cold.

Legs
The long legs are built for speed and also stamina. The wolf can "dog-trot" for hours without tiring.

Jaws
Powerful jaws and large, strong teeth tear flesh and even crack open bones.

Body
The deep chest contains very large lungs and heart, so the wolf does not become short of breath when running long distances.

Tail
The long, bushy tail helps the wolf to balance when running and jumping. Its movements and position—high or low—show the mood and intentions of the wolf to other members of the pack. (Pet dogs do the same with their tails.) Some wolf tails have a black tip.

▲ **An adult gray wolf**

Habitat

Gray wolves are generally found in the wilderness areas of Europe and Asia, as well as in Canada, and several northern U.S. states including Alaska. In all of these places, wolves are very adaptable and occupy many different habitats.

▼ Today wolves live in remote wild areas, keeping well away from towns and humans.

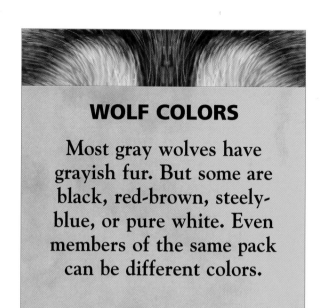

WOLF COLORS

Most gray wolves have grayish fur. But some are black, red-brown, steely-blue, or pure white. Even members of the same pack can be different colors.

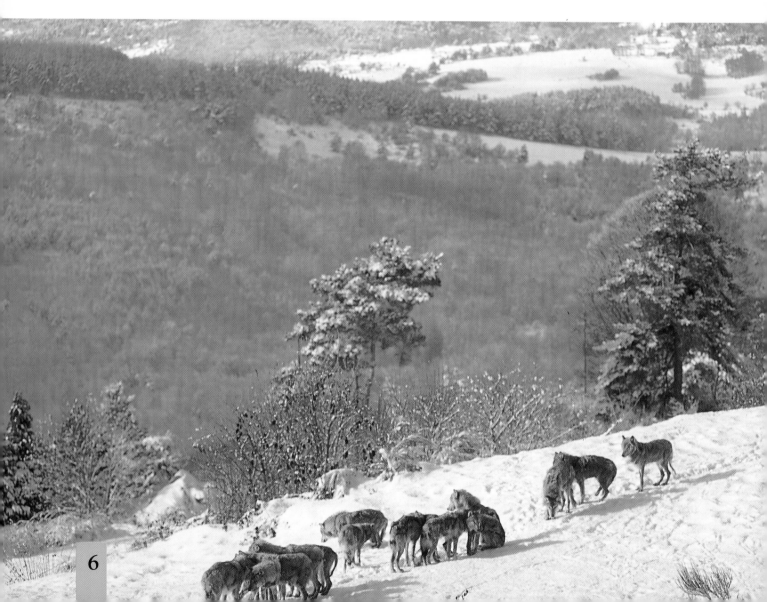

In the United States and Russia, gray wolves live mainly in thick forests. In Italy and Eastern Europe, their home is in the mountains. In northern Canada and Siberia, their habitat is the icy, windy, treeless landscape called the tundra. Yet wolves also live in tropical places such as the scrublands of India and the scorching deserts of Saudi Arabia.

The gray wolf is one of only two kinds, or species, of "true" wolf. The other kind of wolf is the red wolf. There are other types of wolf, such as the maned wolf that lives in South America. Scientists think that maned wolves are not true wolves but distant relatives.

▶ Red wolves once lived in a small region in the southeast United States, but probably became extinct in the wild. Captive-bred red wolves have now been released back into this area in the hope that they will breed and thrive.

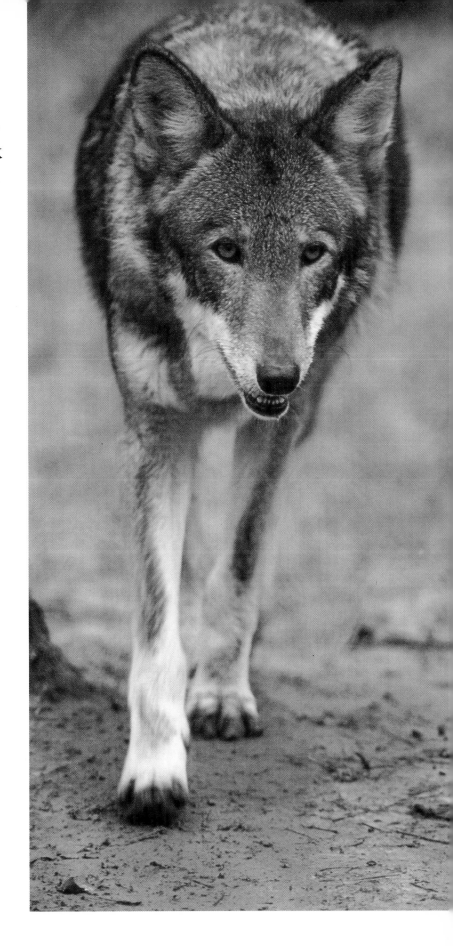

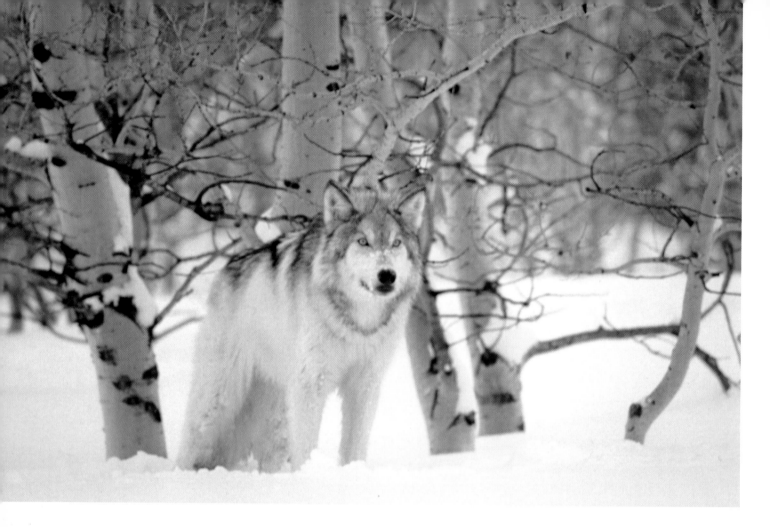

Types of Gray Wolves

Gray wolves from different places and habitats look slightly different. Each of these types is known as a subspecies. The Arctic wolf of the far north is the largest subspecies. Body size is important in the Arctic because larger animals keep in their body heat more effectively than smaller animals. In the bitter cold of the tundra, big animals have a better chance of survival.

Wolves of northern forests are average in size. Those in hot places, such as India, are smaller because they stay cool more efficiently. The smallest wolves live in dry desert areas.

▲ Winters in Canada and northern Europe are long and extremely cold. Wolves spend up to six months a year living in harsh, snowy conditions.

▶ This wolf lives in the Negev Desert in Israel. Like all wolves in hot countries, its fur is much shorter than that of animals living in cold areas further north.

8

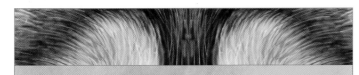

WOLF NAMES

Gray wolves have many other names, depending on their habitat or their fur color.

•

In northern Canada, they are called tundra wolves, Arctic wolves, or white wolves.

•

In most of the United States, they are known as timber wolves.

•

In the southwestern United States and Mexico, they have a local name: lobos.

Wolves are shy and therefore, active mainly at night. They avoid people, so they are rarely seen at close range. Most reports of wolf sightings are really coyotes, jackals, or domestic dogs. A wolf is tall and slender, with big feet and a blunt nose. It is much larger than other wild members of the dog family.

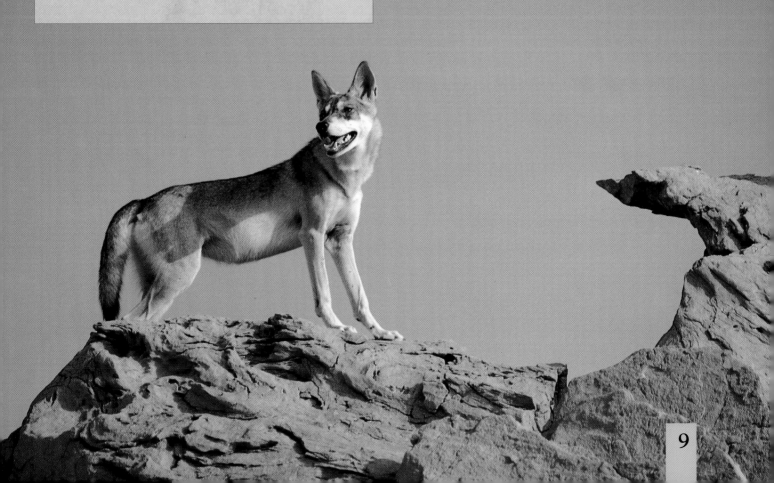

A Wolf Is Born

Inside the gray wolf den, dug deep into the soil, it is even darker than the night outside. A wolf cub is born—the first in a litter of six. As the cubs appear, the mother wolf carefully licks them clean. Each cub uses its sensitive nose to sniff for food. The cubs quickly learn to drink milk from their mother.

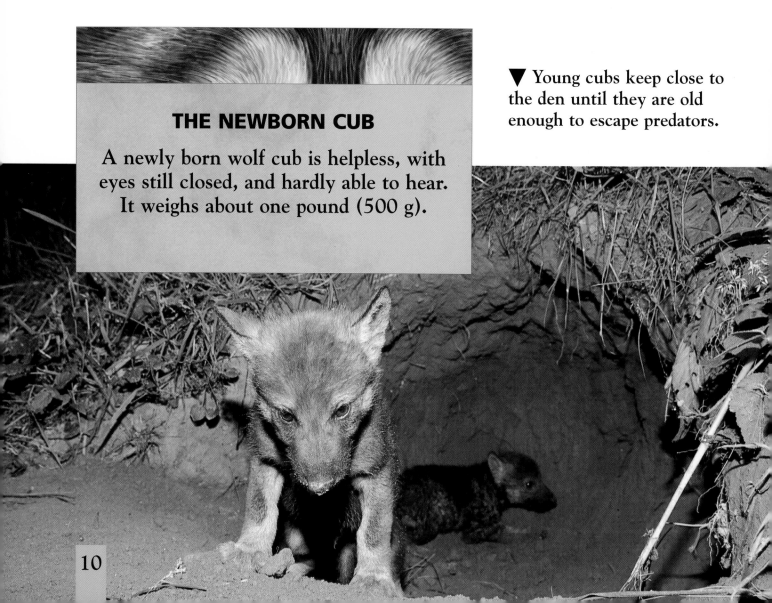

THE NEWBORN CUB

A newly born wolf cub is helpless, with eyes still closed, and hardly able to hear. It weighs about one pound (500 g).

▼ Young cubs keep close to the den until they are old enough to escape predators.

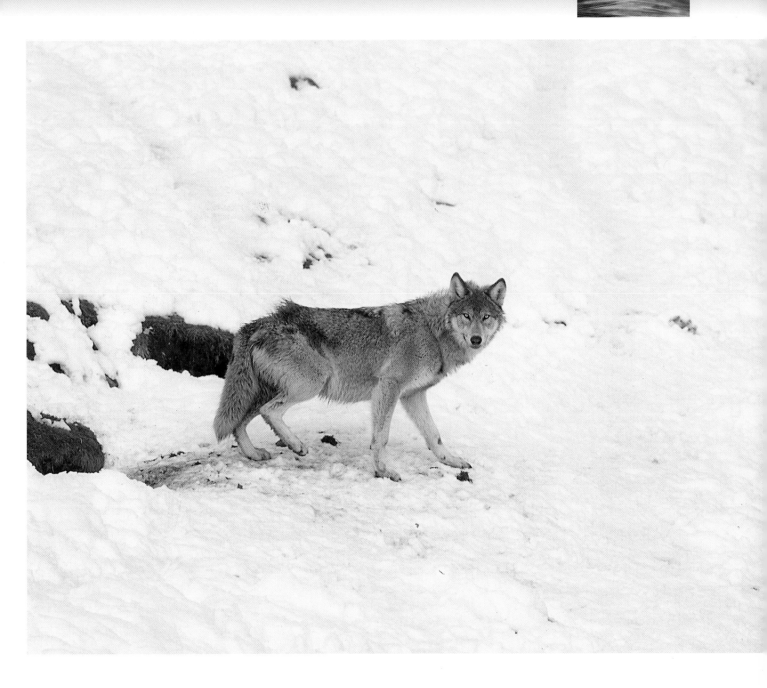

For the first few weeks, the cubs stay in their underground den. They do not leave, even on the rare occasions when their mother goes out. She must stay with them most of the time, because the den is cold and the cubs need the heat from her body. The family sleeps huddled together.

▲ Pack members regularly return to the den to check that the cubs are safe.

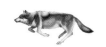

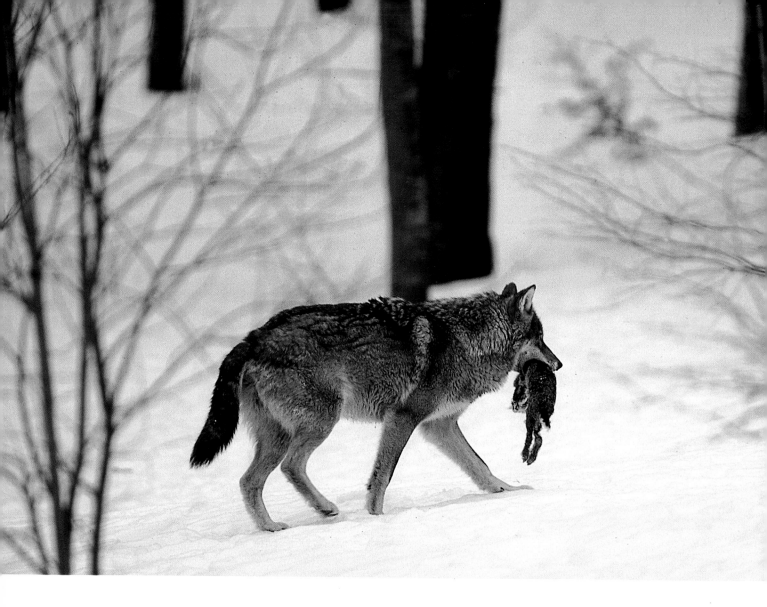

Life in the Den

In the darkness of the den, each gray wolf cub learns to identify its mother and the other cubs by smell. They suckle milk about once every five hours, for a few minutes each time, and grow very quickly. At 12–15 days old, the cubs' eyes open for the first time. One week later they can hear properly, but they are still not ready to go above ground. The mother wolf cannot go off hunting. So other members of the pack bring food back to her, and drop it at the den entrance.

▲ The mother wolf cannot leave her young cubs in the den to go hunting. This wolf from her pack is taking food back to the den.

When the cubs are about one month old they begin to explore the outside world. At first they sit at the den entrance, cautiously look around, and sniff the air. Then the boldest cub steps out, but it does not go far and suddenly darts back to the safety of its mother. As the cubs grow older, they gradually become more and more confident. They spend more time exploring, and learn their way around the nearby area by sight and scent.

▼ Deep under ground the cubs can smell the world outside. They soon become curious and leave the den to look around.

THE WOLF DEN

The entrance to a typical den is about 24 inches (60 cm) across. It leads into a tunnel that can be up to 30 feet (9 m) deep. At the end is a large chamber where the cubs are born. The cubs stay in or near the den until they are about 8 weeks old.

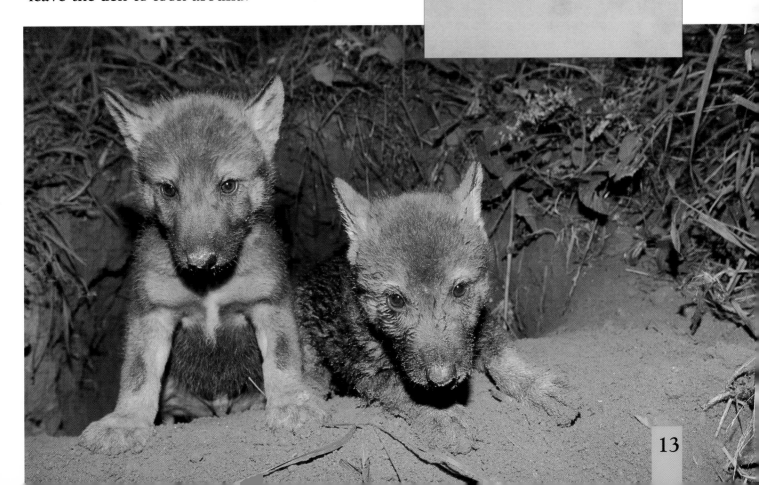

Meeting the Pack

The adults of the gray wolf pack can smell and hear the cubs in the den. They often stand at the den entrance, listening and sniffing, but a sharp growl from the cubs' mother stops them from coming in.

When the youngsters appear for the first time, the pack gathers around. The adults lie nearby as the cubs tumble and play. The boldest cubs climb onto them and bite their ears, noses, and tails. These activities introduce the cubs to the pack. The survival of every wolf depends on identifying members of its own pack.

▼ When they first leave the den, young cubs stay very close together until they are confident enough to explore alone.

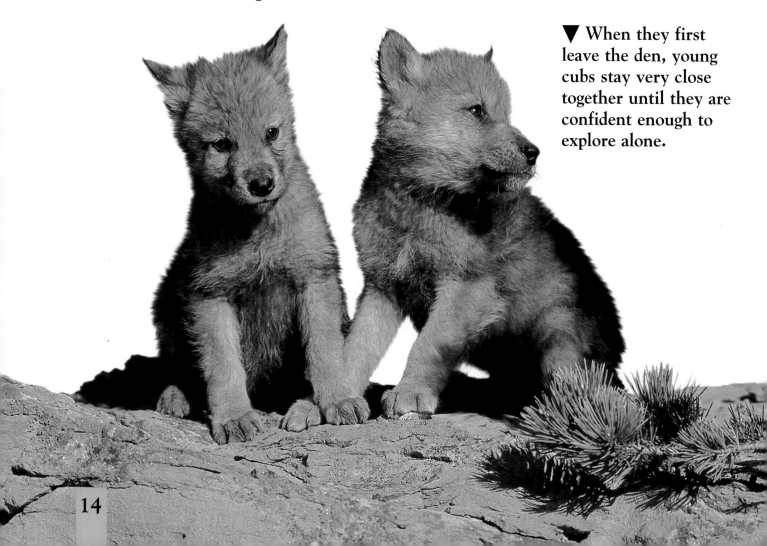

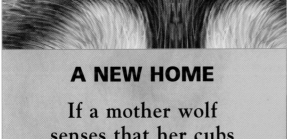

A NEW HOME

If a mother wolf senses that her cubs are in danger, she will pick them up in her mouth, one by one, and carry them to a new den. This can be a long distance away, even several miles from the original den.

▼ Young cubs completely relax when picked up in their mother's mouth. This makes them much easier to carry.

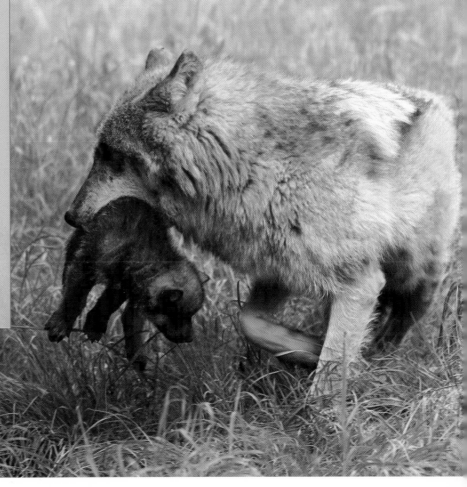

The cub's teeth appear when it is about one month old. They are small but sharp. The adults usually put up with the cubs, but move away if the games get too rough. Soon the cubs begin to play-fight among themselves, with snarls and growls. This is the start of a lifelong battle to become the leader of the pack.

Learning to Survive

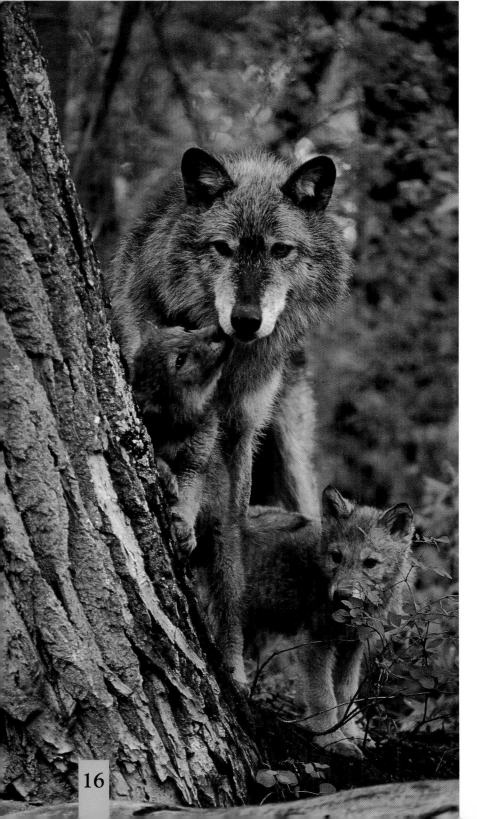

At about four weeks of age, the gray wolf cubs begin to eat meat and other solid foods. They still take mother's milk, but the adults in the pack bring them meals. If an adult catches prey near the den, it carries the food back in its mouth, and the cubs practice tearing it apart. The biggest and strongest male cub usually gets the first bite.

◀ Wolves with young cubs are always on the lookout for predators that might be happy to make a meal of them.

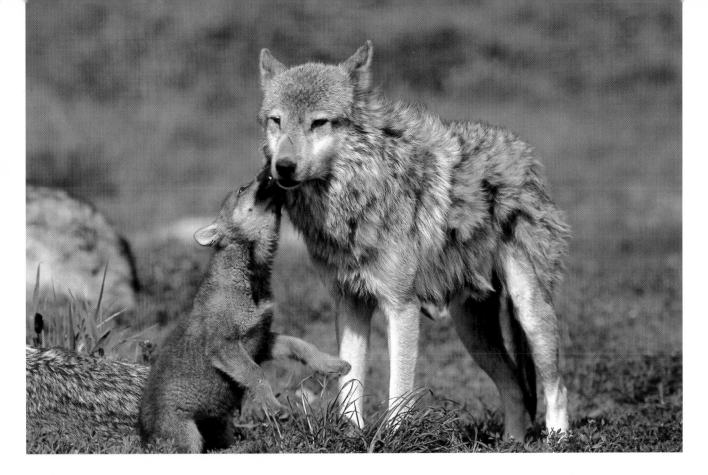

▲ Cubs can smell when an adult brings food to the den, even when it is inside the stomach. The scent of meat makes the cubs beg frantically.

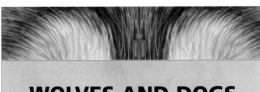

WOLVES AND DOGS

If a wolf meets a domestic (pet) dog, the outcome is not certain. They might slink away to avoid a battle, or sometimes they might get into a fight. Occasionally, if one is a male and the other is a female, the two may mate and produce young.

To carry food over longer distances, a wolf swallows chunks into its stomach. This makes traveling easier and keeps the meat warm and free from dirt. On return, the cubs smell the meal. They beg by licking the adult's mouth. The meat is not yet digested, and with a short coughing action, the adult regurgitates (vomits) the food onto the ground. Again, the strongest cub is first in line. If another cub comes too close, he may start a fight.

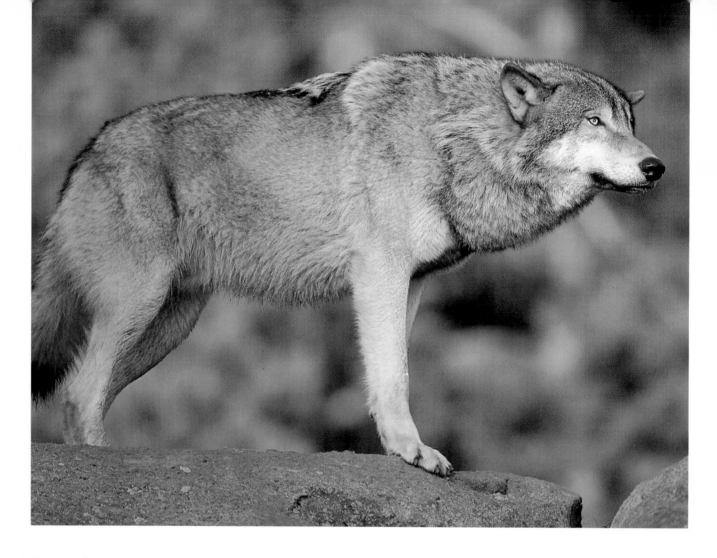

On Their Own

Young gray wolf cubs need to mix with the adults. They supply food and also teach the cubs how to communicate and show their intentions. Wolves do this in many ways. They use body postures, such as pulling back their ears or cocking them forward. They also use sounds such as whines, yaps, snarls, and growls.

As the cubs grow, they are less troubled by the cold weather. Their mother can leave the den and join the hunt, but another adult usually stays behind in case of danger, such as a bear or a rival wolf pack.

▲ With head down, ears held flat, and tail between his legs, this wolf is showing the "submissive" pose. This is a sign that he completely accepts the authority of the pack leaders.

IMPORTANCE OF SMELL

A wolf's most important sense is smell. Pack members recognize each other, and cubs recognize their mother, mainly by scent. Hunting wolves follow the smell of prey for many miles, often hours after the prey has passed.

Waiting at the Den

When the mother wolf trots away for the first time, the cubs follow, but they are nervous out in the open and soon dash back to their den. The pack is away hunting for many hours, and the cubs whine for their mother. When she returns, they rush to meet her, and she licks them. After she brings up food for them, she settles down to sleep.

▼ Mother and cubs lick each other as a sign of affection.

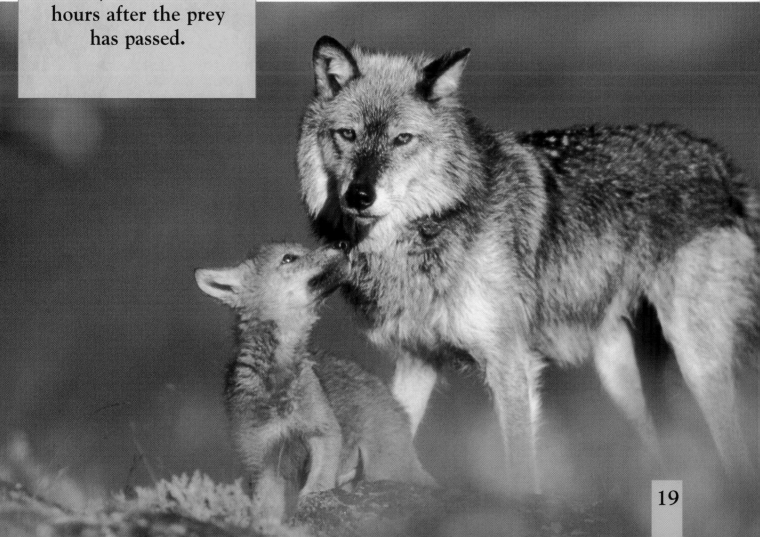

Leaving the Den

The cubs spend their days sleeping and playing with each other. They begin to practice the skills that they will need for survival. A cub will stalk and pounce on the others, grab them with sharp teeth, hold tight, and shake them hard. They rarely harm each other. Instead, this play-fighting strengthens their muscles and sharpens their reactions.

▼ Playing builds up the cubs' muscles and sharpens their senses.

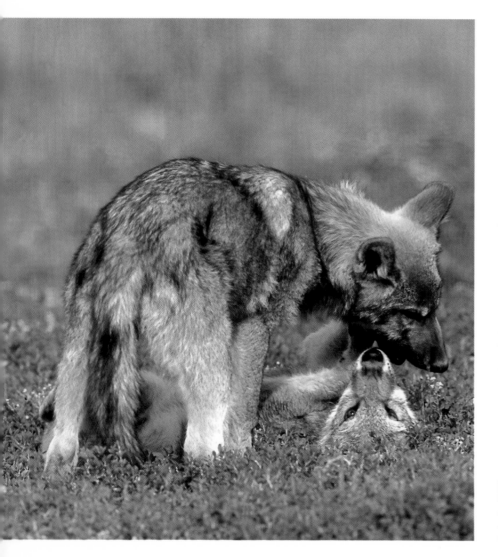

Around the den are many old bones, carried in by the adults. The meat was eaten long ago, but the cubs gnaw and chew at them. At eight weeks old they are completely weaned. They have stopped taking milk from their mother and rely entirely on solid foods. For the last time, the litter of cubs leaves the den.

▶ Play gets rougher as the cubs get bigger. They often have violent fights over food.

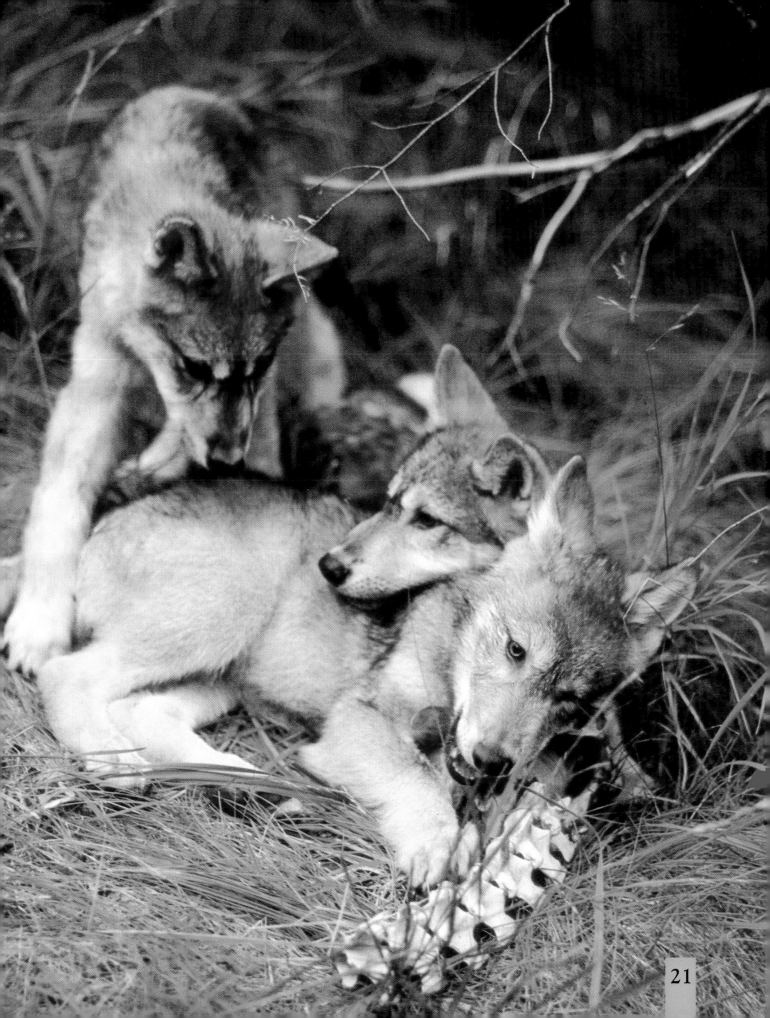

Joining the Pack

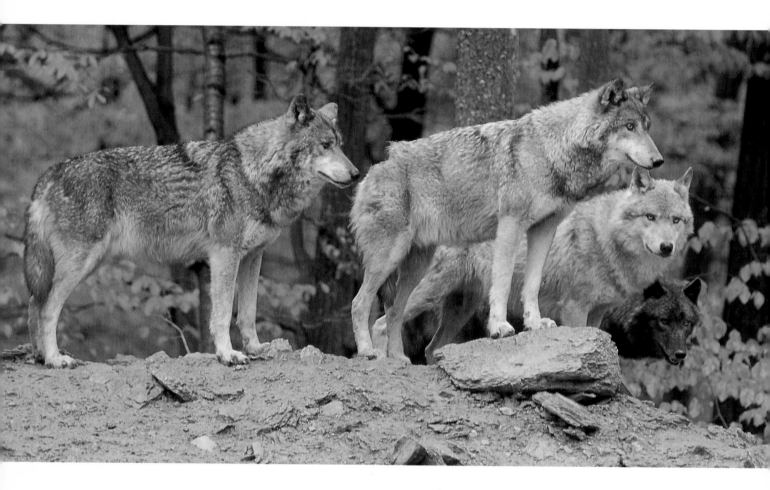

As the gray wolf cubs leave their den for the last time, their mother leads them to a rendezvous area. This is a place where the whole pack gathers. It is usually on an open, grassy mound, with views all around. It is the central place for the pack's activities. The plants are trampled by wolves walking and lying, bones are scattered around, and there are shallow holes that older cubs have dug as they played.

▲ Wolves are at their most efficient when they act together as a pack. Lone wolves have difficulty finding a territory and are less likely to catch large prey.

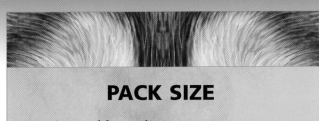

PACK SIZE

A wolf pack varies in size from only two to more than fifteen members. In large wilderness areas, most packs contain between four and seven adults, plus a few cubs. In small forests there may just be one female, one male, and their cubs.

▼ Cubs will beg food from any member of the pack.

The cubs are now two months old. They can follow the adults for nearly a mile, but they are not big enough to take part in a hunt. They stay in the rendezvous area while the adults are away. After a hunt, the whole pack returns to feed and play with the cubs. If they have killed a large animal, they bring back extra pieces of meat and bury them nearby. They can dig up the hidden pieces later.

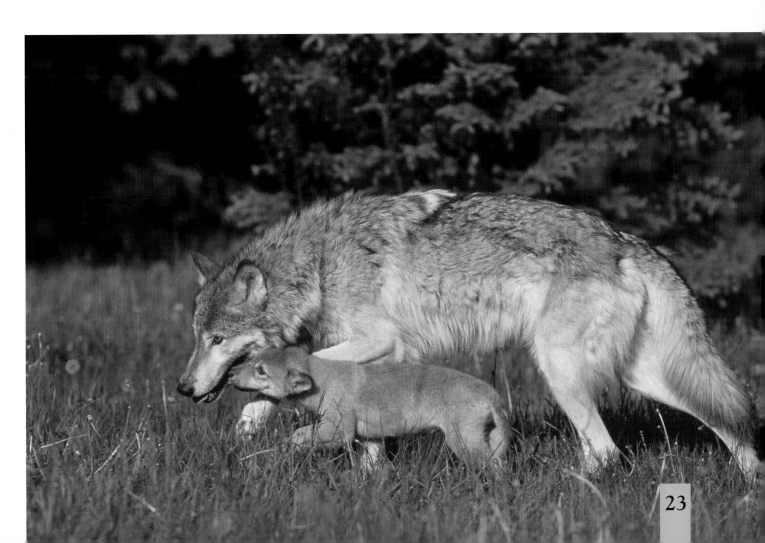

Sleeping and Exploring

The gray wolf cubs now sleep above ground, like the adults. During warm weather, they lie on their side. When it rains, they curl up and put their nose under the end of their bushy tail to keep it warm. Their feet also lose heat quickly, so they tuck them beneath their body. In a blizzard, they can be covered in snow yet warm in their thick fur.

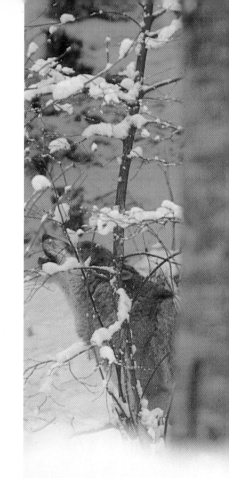

▼ This wolf cub is about four months old.

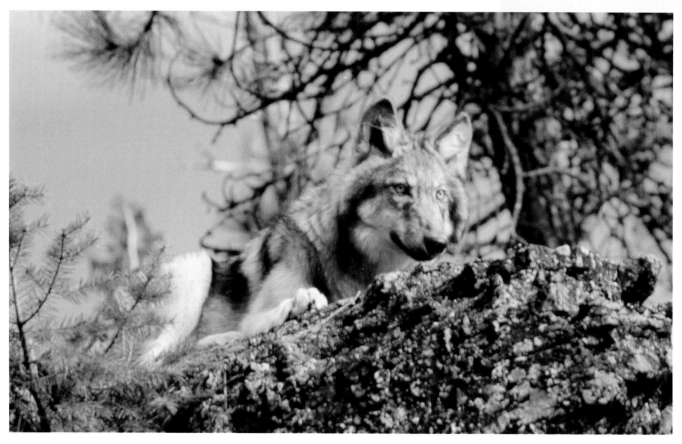

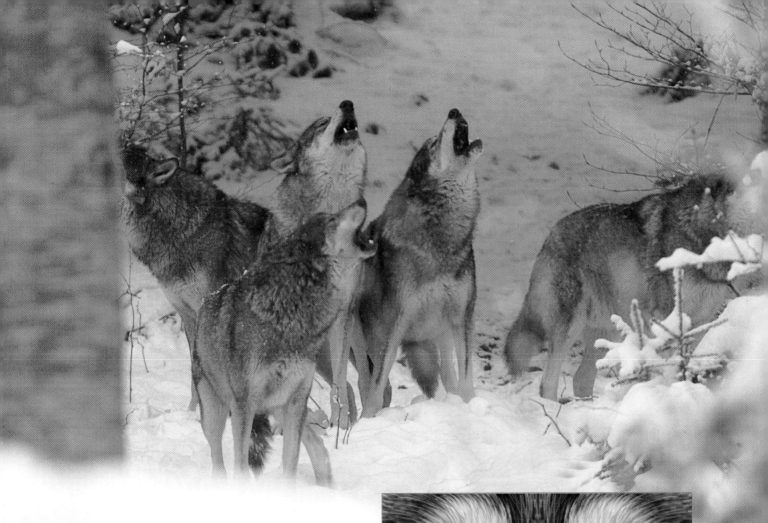

▲ The distant sound of howling is often the only clue that wolves live nearby.

At six months old, the cubs weigh about 67 pounds (25 kg). They play together less and spend more time alone. The cubs explore the rendezvous area, hunting small prey like mice and other rodents. The adults still bring them meat. At about eight months old, the cubs are ready to go on a real hunt with the rest of the pack.

HOWLING WOLF

Howls are one type of sound that wolves use to communicate. Each wolf howls for only about five seconds, but when the whole pack joins in, the calls become mingled and seem much longer. Howls help pack members to keep together, and ward off nearby rival packs.

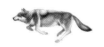

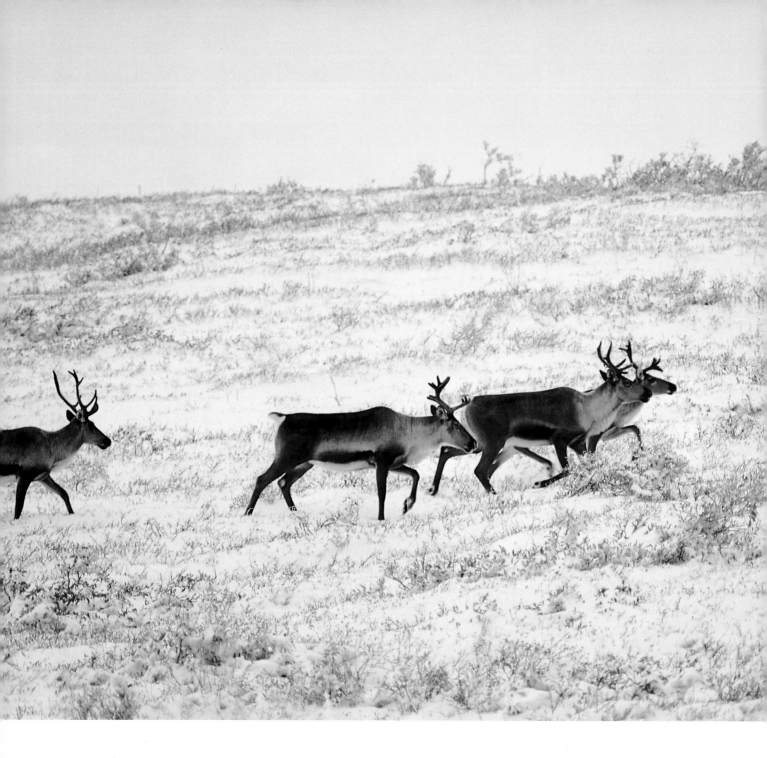

Pack on the Move

A wolf pack is usually on the move, searching for prey. Packs that live in the Arctic follow the caribou (a type of deer) that travel, or migrate, long distances to find fresh grazing. Caribou are the main food for these wolf packs.

▲ Caribou make up an important part of the diet of wolves that live in the Arctic.

A wolf pack lives and hunts in a huge patch of land known as its territory. Wolves living in woods and forests usually stay in one small territory all year. Their prey do not migrate. Pack members patrol their territory regularly to keep out rival wolves. They mark the boundaries with strong-smelling urine that tells other wolves to keep away.

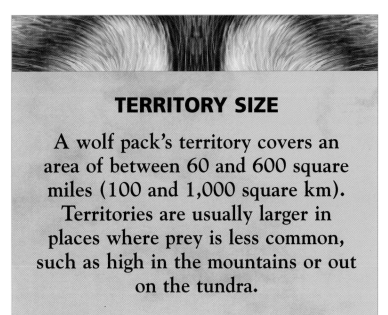

TERRITORY SIZE

A wolf pack's territory covers an area of between 60 and 600 square miles (100 and 1,000 square km). Territories are usually larger in places where prey is less common, such as high in the mountains or out on the tundra.

Sometimes rival wolves move into a territory that is already occupied by a pack. The resident pack becomes restless and aggressive, and tries to drive out the invaders. There may be a fight. The cubs are not safe during these territorial battles. Some of the younger, weaker wolves can be badly hurt or even killed.

▶ This male wolf is scent-marking a tree by spraying it with his urine.

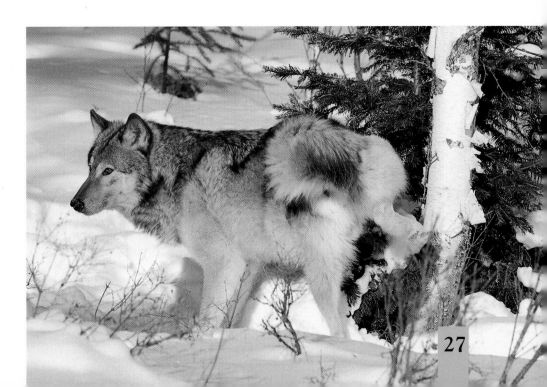

Adult Life

A young male gray wolf will be ready to mate with a female at three years of age. However, he may never get the chance. In each pack, only one male and one female breed to produce cubs. They are known as the alpha pair. Alphas are the leaders of the pack.

If a young male wolf stays with his pack, one day he may have to challenge the alpha male, or wait for him to die. Then he can become the alpha male himself. If he is small or weak, he might never breed. Small adult wolves spend their lives helping to feed and protect the cubs of the alpha pair, for the good of the whole pack.

▼ The way a wolf behaves depends on its position within the pack. Each wolf must know which animals are weaker and which are stronger. This affects its choice of food and its chances of breeding.

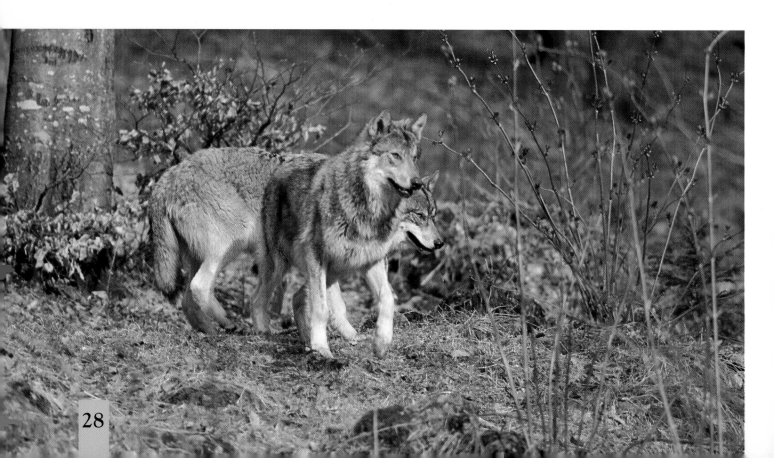

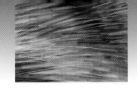

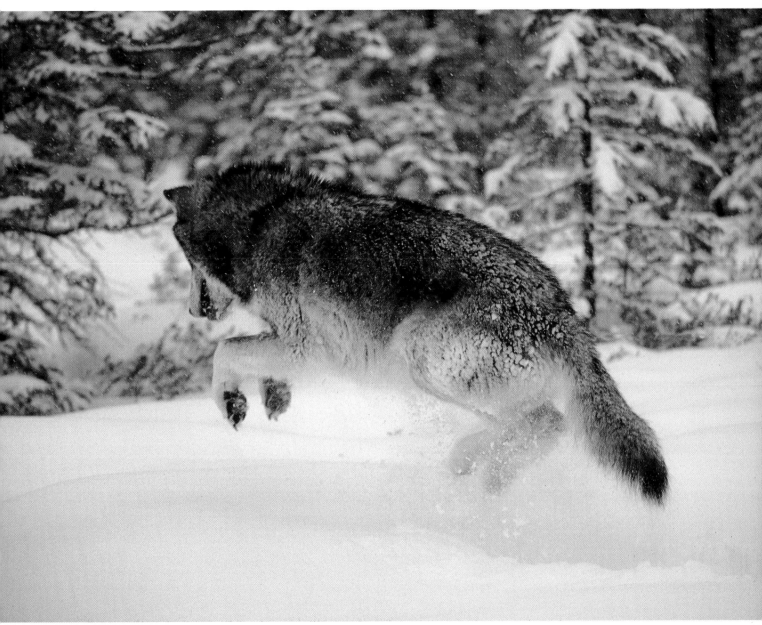

▲ This lone wolf is having to hunt its own food. It is pouncing on a mouse.

Another choice is to leave the pack and try elsewhere. Wolves who leave their original packs are called dispersers. For weeks a disperser travels, hunting for his own food. Then he meets another disperser, and another. Soon several come together, and they begin a new pack.

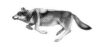

Leaders of the Pack

In a new pack, the young male gray wolves compete with one another. After a few tussles, the biggest and strongest wolf becomes the alpha male. In these battles, the larger and healthier wolf usually wins by snarling at rivals, but if two wolves are equally matched, they fight. Fights are mostly just a test of strength. The loser retreats before injuries occur. Deaths are very rare.

▼ Low-ranking wolves sometimes beg food from the pack leaders. This is a signal that they accept the dominance of the alpha pair.

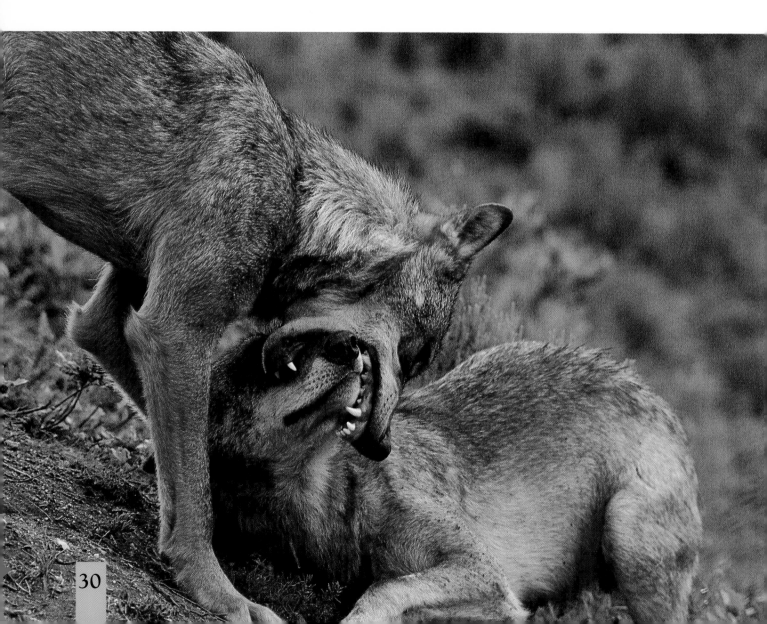

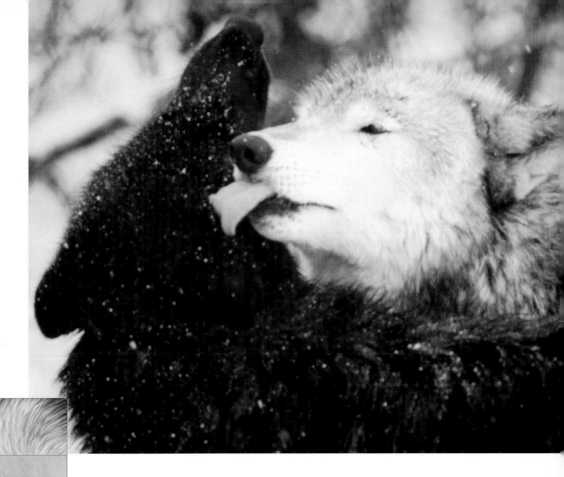

▶ The alpha pair spend a lot of time licking each other and sleeping close together.

WOLF BREEDING

The wolf mating season is usually February and March, and the cubs are born after about 62 days. A female can have up to 14 cubs in one litter, but the usual number is 6 or 7. There is only one litter of cubs each year. This means a female may produce 45 cubs during her lifetime.

Separate battles sort out which wolf will be the alpha female. The alpha male and alpha female take charge of their group. Over a period of about four weeks in early spring, the alpha pair are rarely apart. They travel and rest together, lick each other, and mate many times.

The alpha female chooses her breeding den. She may use an old den, a cave, or a rocky shelter. More often, she digs a tunnel with her strong front paws. At the end she makes a chamber just wide enough for her to lie down, ready for her cubs.

Hunting

The new gray wolf pack must challenge other packs in the area to establish a territory. During the day, they rest in their rendezvous area. They become active just before sunset. Wolves hunt mainly at night, when it is cooler in hot regions and they can sneak up on victims in the darkness.

▼ Wolves track prey by scent. They can follow a smell even in deep snow.

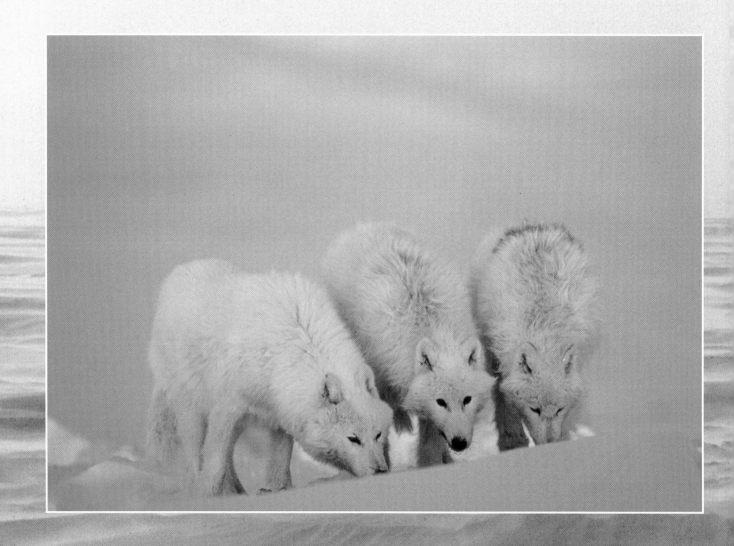

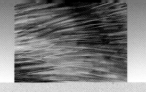

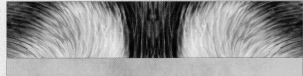

WOLF-TROT

Wolves usually "dog-trot" at about 5 miles (8 km) per hour. They can travel all day and all night at this speed. During an attack they can race along at almost 37 miles (60 km) per hour, but only for a minute or so, over a distance of about half a mile.

Wolves find their prey by their main sense—smell. They can travel 15 miles (30 km) or more in a single night to reach food. One wolf hunting by itself can catch a rabbit or hare. But when six wolves work together, they can bring down prey heavier than all of their weights added together, such as moose and elk.

▼ Wolves need to eat more in cold weather, when prey is usually more difficult to find.

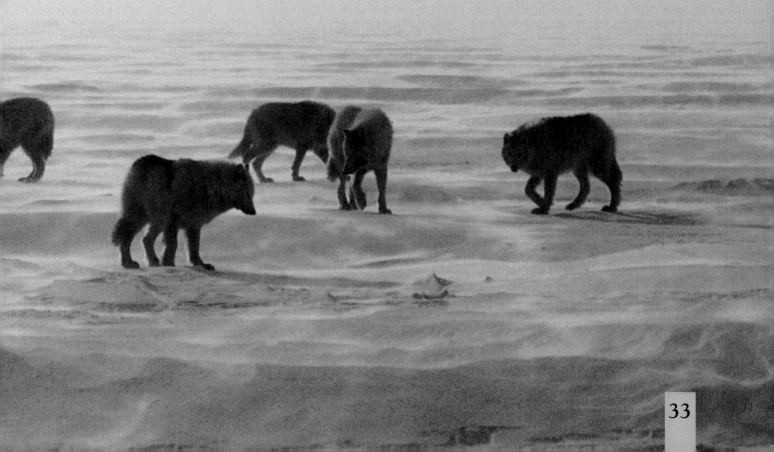

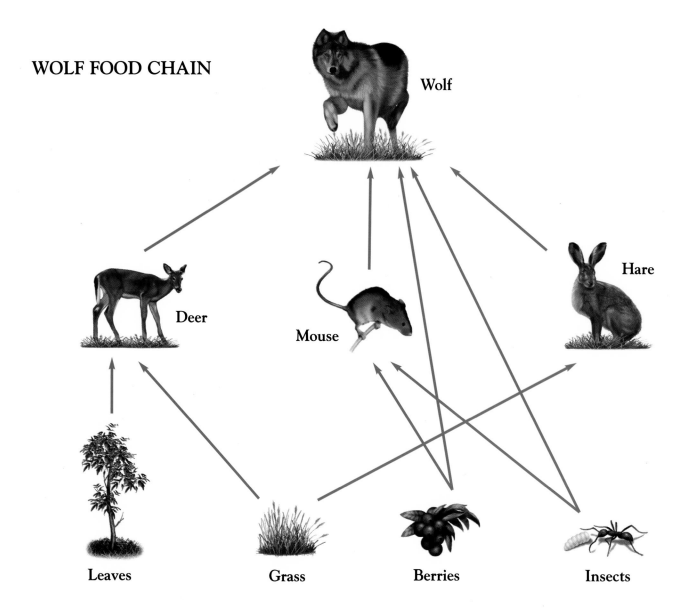

WOLF FOOD CHAIN

Wolf

Hare

Deer

Mouse

Leaves

Grass

Berries

Insects

Closing In for the Kill

When wolves come across a herd of deer, they will pick out deer that are slower or weaker than others. The wolves test them with a series of quick attacks. If a deer runs off quickly at high speed, the wolves do not waste time chasing. They try another. Once the wolves have found a herd member that is old, ill, weak, young, or injured, they close in.

▲ Wolves are at the top of their food chain. Their prey depends upon their habitat. Wolves in deserts hunt different animals than those that live in the Arctic.

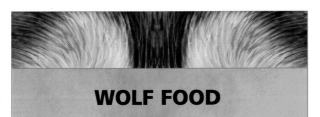

WOLF FOOD

Wolves are mainly carnivores. They kill and eat other animals. A pack can catch large animals such as deer and wild sheep. A single wolf hunts small prey such as mice and rabbits. In times of food shortage, wolves can eat insects, fish, birds, eggs, fruits, berries, and carrion (dead animals).

The younger wolves try to drive the chosen deer toward the large adults. Then the pack attempts to form a circle around the animal. As the deer turns to run, one of the alpha pair darts in and grabs its back leg or its nose, to prevent escape. The others charge in and grab a piece of the victim. In a few seconds, the deer is dead.

▼ Wolves are always hungry in the coldest days of winter. At this time even a fully-grown deer will feed the pack for just a few days.

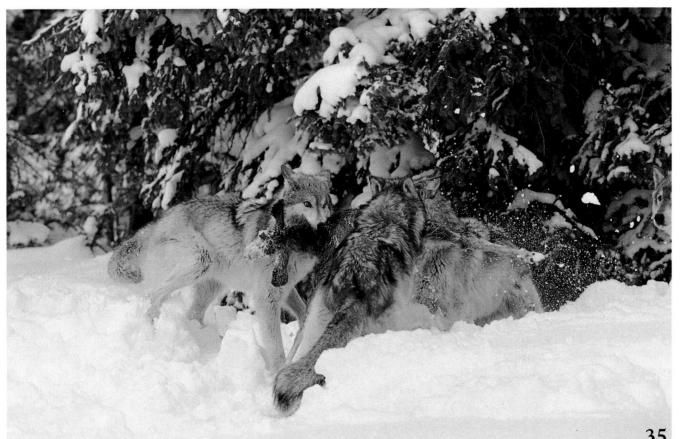

Sharing the Meal

After a big kill, the alpha pair of gray wolves have first choice of food. They usually go for soft, nutritious parts of the victim, such as the heart and liver. The others fight for their shares. They snarl, growl, and snap at each other.

▼ Low-ranking wolves must wait until the alpha pair have fed before they can begin to eat.

WOLF APPETITE

A 130-pound (50-kg) wolf can eat 40 pounds (15 kg) of food in a single day. This is almost one-third of its own body weight. Wolves do this because they are not always successful in the hunt. Many days they eat nothing at all.

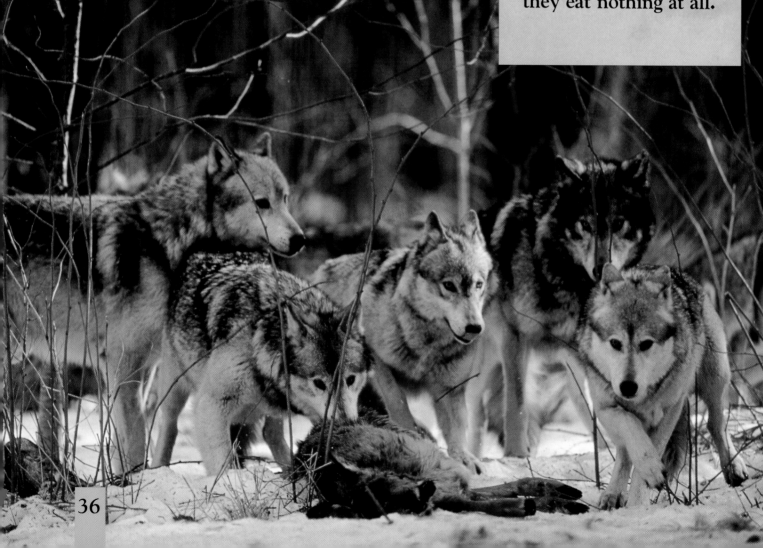

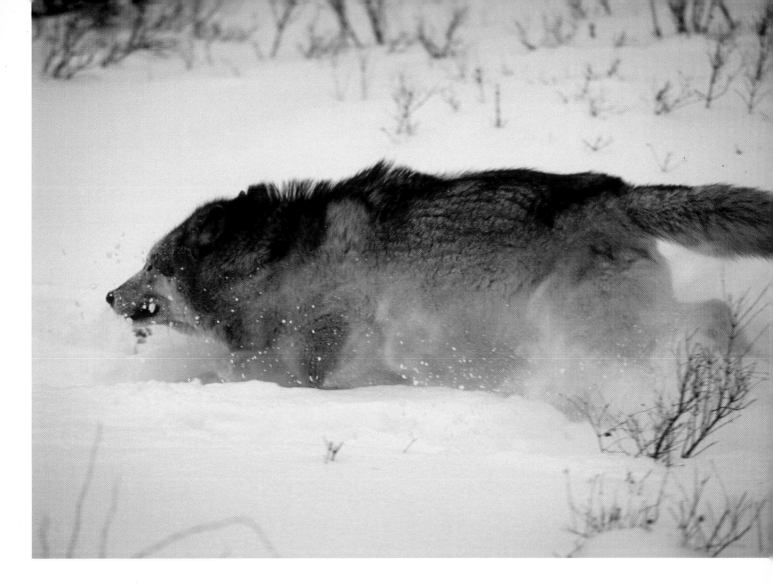

▲ Hunting is difficult in winter. Wolves find it hard to run fast in deep snow. Prey animals can also easily see the wolves' dark fur against the white surroundings.

When the pack has caught a large animal, every wolf can eat its fill and there will still be meat left over. This remaining food is often buried in the ground. In times when prey is scarce, the pack can always return and dig up the food.

A wolf that hunts alone usually crouches low to the ground. It creeps toward the prey, as close as possible. When the prey senses the approaching danger, it runs, and the wolf immediately follows. If the wolf does not catch up to the prey within a minute or two, it turns away and tries another target.

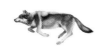

Wolves and People

In myth and legend, wolves are usually monsters. They attack villages and carry off children. They are cunning and evil in stories such as *Little Red Riding Hood* and *Three Little Pigs*. Werewolves are said to be half-human, half-wolf creatures that howl at the full moon.

Wolves are supposed to be vicious, bloodthirsty killers that attack humans on sight, but this image is not true. The myth has grown because people misunderstand wolves, and because—throughout history—wolves have occasionally killed farmers' livestock.

▼ In the Middle Ages many people in Europe believed in werewolves. These were thought to be humans that changed into half-wolf and attacked both people and animals.

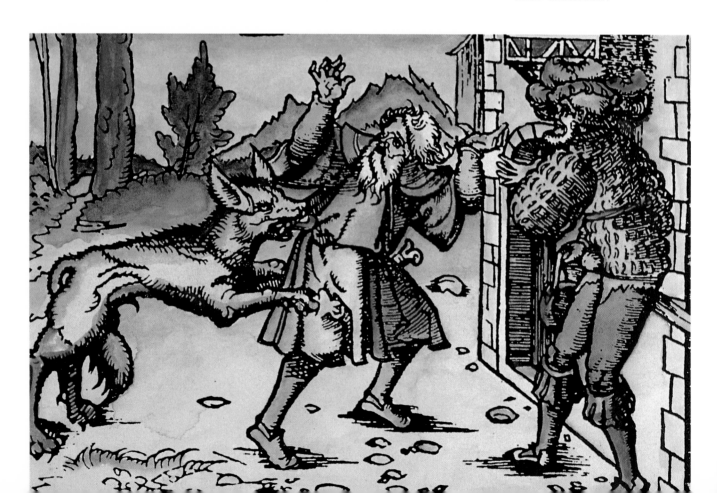

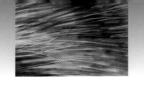

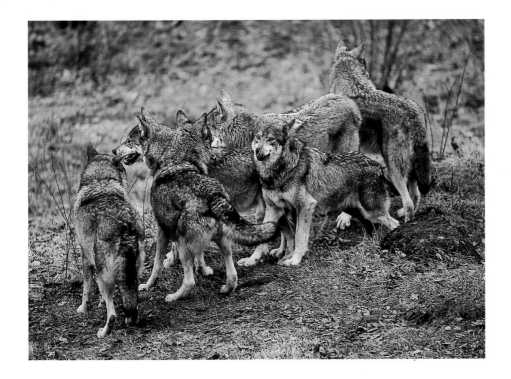

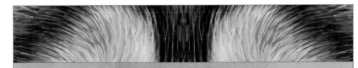

◀ This wolf pack in Germany is one of the few that still survives in western Europe.

The truth is that gray wolves are very wary and take great care to avoid people. Attacks on humans are extremely rare. They usually happen only when a wolf is starving or diseased.

Even so, people have hunted wolves for centuries. About 800 years ago in Great Britain, some farmers had to pay rent to the local landowner in the form of wolf skins. This made sure many wolves were killed. The last British wolf died in 1743.

WOLF TO DOG

Wild wolf cubs were probably captured and somewhat tamed by people at least 11,000 years ago. Over time they grew more tame, and were bred to help with hunting, guarding, and being companions. Gradually these wild gray wolves became domesticated dogs. Every size, shape, and color of pet dog in the world has the wolf as its distant ancestor.

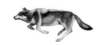

Wolves in North America

Long ago in North America, native people respected and admired gray wolves. But European settlers brought with them an ancient, deep fear of the animal, and soon started killing them. Wolves became the most widely hunted animal in American history. By the beginning of the 20th century, they were nearly extinct. Yet the government still paid rewards of up to $50 for each wolf shot, trapped, poisoned, or somehow killed. Wolves were soon wiped out from most parts of the United States.

The slaughter was nothing new. Gray wolves had been treated in this way in almost every country where they lived. Farmers and ranchers believe that wolf packs kill many farm animals. But raids on farms are far from common. Wolves distrust us and our smells. They prefer remote wilderness areas that are not used for farming.

▼ Even today wolves in North America and elsewhere are illegally killed by poachers.

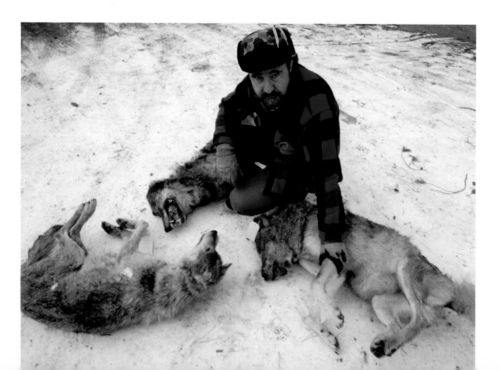

► These wolves are found in the Abruzzi National Park in Italy. They live quite close to mountain villages, but they have learned to be extremely wary of people. Packs are rarely seen and take great care to avoid contact with humans.

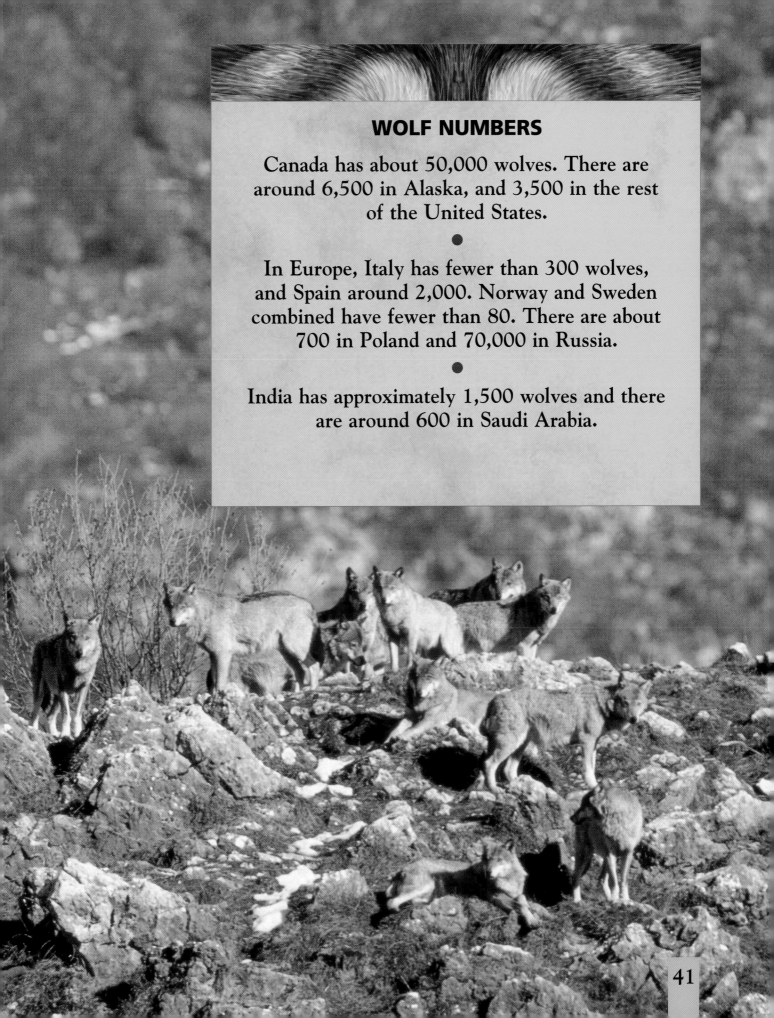

WOLF NUMBERS

Canada has about 50,000 wolves. There are around 6,500 in Alaska, and 3,500 in the rest of the United States.

•

In Europe, Italy has fewer than 300 wolves, and Spain around 2,000. Norway and Sweden combined have fewer than 80. There are about 700 in Poland and 70,000 in Russia.

•

India has approximately 1,500 wolves and there are around 600 in Saudi Arabia.

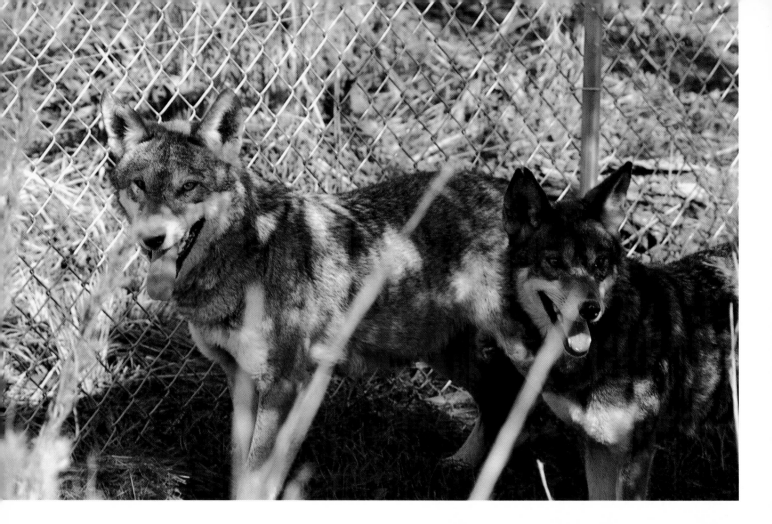

▲ These wolves in the United States were born in captivity, but they are about to be released into the wild for the first time in their lives.

Saving Wolves

In recent years, our view of the gray wolf has changed. We understand more about this creature and know that it rarely poses a threat to people. Many countries have begun conservation efforts to save wild wolves. In most of western Europe, laws now protect wolves from hunting and trapping.

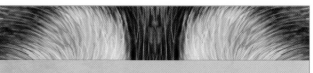

AMAZING JOURNEY

Gray wolves cover enormous distances as they hunt, patrol their territories, and care for their cubs. During its lifetime, a wolf probably travels farther than any other land mammal on earth—apart from, perhaps, the caribou it hunts, and the human.

▼ A scientist is attaching a radio collar to a wild wolf that has been shot with a dart gun. The wolf will sleep for a few minutes before running off. Scientists will then be able to follow the wolf's movement by tracking the radio signal transmitted by the collar.

In the United States, apart from the state of Alaska, the wolf is now an endangered species. The U.S. Fish and Wildlife Service has captured wild wolves in British Columbia and Alberta, and transported them back to large nature areas such as Yellowstone National Park and central Idaho, where they once lived. The wolves have bred and increased in numbers. There are now several well-established packs. The future for North American wolves looks brighter.

Sadly, even today, a few countries hang onto their old beliefs. Wolves are still being killed there, for no good reason.

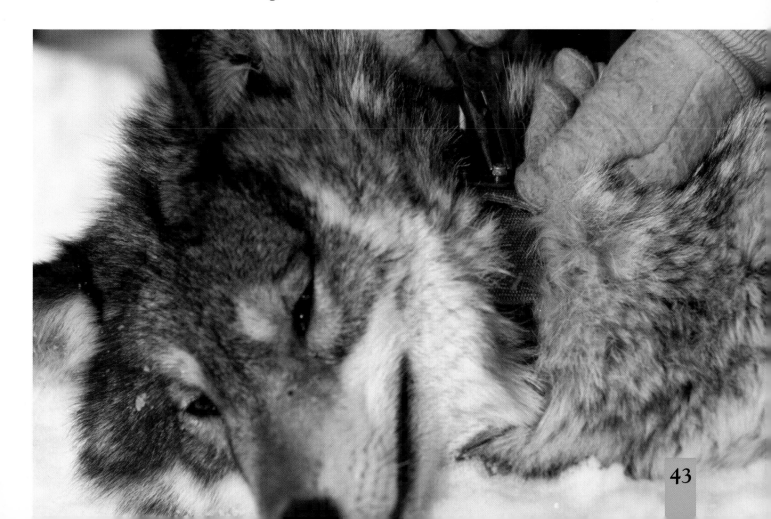

Wolf Life Cycle

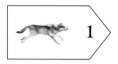 **1** The newborn gray wolf cub is helpless and unable to see or hear. It weighs around 17 ounces (500 g). An average litter of cubs is 6–7, rarely 12 or more.

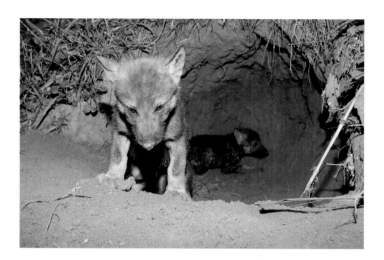

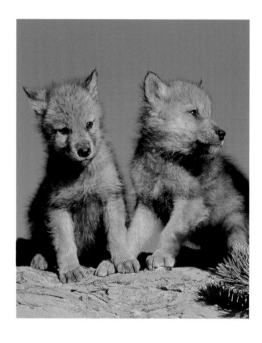

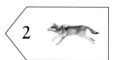 **2** The cub's eyes open by 12–15 days. At 3–4 weeks old, it leaves the underground den for the first time. The cub meets other members of its pack and learns to communicate with them.

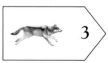 **3** The cub learns sounds such as yelps, howls, and snarls, and body postures such as bared teeth, flattened ears, crouching down, and holding the tail up or down. It takes its place as junior pack member.

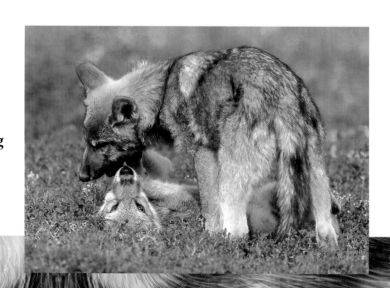

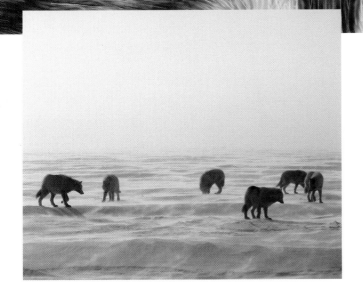

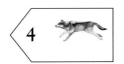 **4** At eight months old, the cub weighs around 67 pounds (25 kg). It is fast and strong enough to hunt with the others. The pack moves from one rendezvous site to another. Sites are often 5–6 miles (8–10 km) apart.

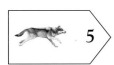 **5** Female wolves can breed at about two years of age, and males by three years. But both usually have to wait until they are strong enough to beat rivals and become the alpha pair. They may leave to join another pack, or form a new one.

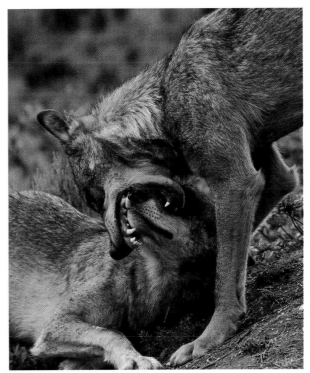

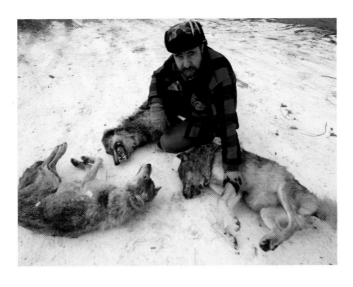

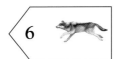 **6** Less than half of newborn wolf cubs reach adulthood. In the wild, average adult life span is around 10 years. Most adult wolves die of starvation or old age. Their occasional enemies include bears, wolverines, large cats such as cougars, and rival wolf packs. Their only serious threat is us.

Glossary

Alpha pair (AL-fuh pair) The chief male and female wolves in a pack, and the only ones that have cubs.

Breed To produce young.

Carnivore (KAR-nuh-vor) An animal that eats mainly flesh or meat.

Carrion (KA-ree-on) The remains or leftovers of a dead animal.

Endangered (en-DAYN-jurd) Living things that are low in numbers and are at risk of dying out altogether (becoming extinct).

Habitat (HAB-uh-tat) The natural place for an animal or plant.

Litter (LIT-ur) A group of young animals born at the same time to the same mother. They are brothers and sisters.

Predator (PRED-uh-tur) An animal that hunts and kills other creatures.

Prey A creature that is killed and eaten by another animal.

Rendezvous area (RON-day-voo AIR-ee-uh) The place where a wolf pack meets. Rendezvous is another word for a meeting.

Scrubland (SKRUHB-land) An open area of land where shrubs, small trees, and grass grow together.

Suckle (SUHK-uhl) To drink milk from a mother mammal's teats.

Territory (TER-uh-tor-ee) An area that is controlled and defended by an animal or group of animals.

Tundra (TUHN-druh) A type of landscape with low plants, bogs, and grasses, in the far north of the world.

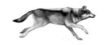

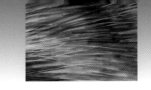

Further Information

Organizations to Contact

World Wildlife Fund-U.S.
1250 24th Street, N.W.
Washington, D.C. 20037
Tel: (202) 293-4800

Wolf Education and Research Center
P.O. Box 217
Winchester, ID 83555
Tel: (208) 924-6960

Books to Read

Greenaway, Theresa. *The Secret World of: Wolves, Wild Dogs, and Foxes*. New York: Raintree Steck-Vaughn Publishers, 2001.

Lopez, Barry. *Of Wolves and Men*. New York: Scribner, 1982.

Mech, L. David. *The Way of the Wolf*. Stillwater, MN: Voyager Press, 1995.

Simon, Seymour. *Wolves*. New York: HarperTrophy, 1995.

Index

Page numbers in **bold** refer to photographs or illustrations.

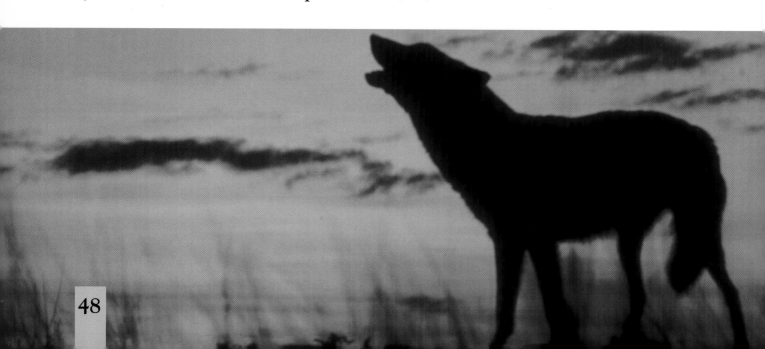